My Fertility Journey

My Fertility Journey

EXPECT, POSITION AND ENDURE

Deanna Townsend-Smith Ed.D.

ISBN: 1977697356
ISBN 13: 9781977697356
Library of Congress Control Number: 2017915043
CreateSpace Independent Publishing Platform
North Charleston, South Carolina

Dedication

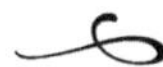

Dedicated to my Husband, Son, and those I carried but never knew.

Rejection

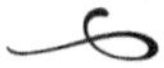

Research from the Centers for Disease Control and Prevention (2017) indicates that 6 percent of women, men, and couples experience some difficulty achieving pregnancy within one year of trying. You hear about couples experiencing fertility issues and feel bad for them, but you never imagine yourself in that group until it happens to you. While the percentage seems low, imagine being among that 6 percent. What effect would it have on you?

I felt that my body rejected what it was supposed to do—not once, but repeatedly. When I married my husband in 2001, I never thought we'd be in that 6 percent. Yet three years later, we weren't successful in achieving pregnancy. As a health-conscious person, I visited my ob-gyn yearly, as recommended, and began initial conversations about our lack of success at pregnancy. At first, the doctor dismissed this conversation until I began to advocate for myself. A test to evaluate my fallopian tubes determined there was no blockage. After further examination, the doctor discovered that I had fibroid tumors.

Considering the fibroid tumors and the poignant fact that we had gone three years without conceiving, the ob-gyn recommended removing the fibroids and preserving my fertility through a procedure called a myomectomy. I proceeded with the surgery during the summer of 2004, fortunate to work in the education field and to have the summer to recuperate for the required six weeks. The doctor assured me that after the procedure, our chances of conceiving would be higher, as he firmly believed (at the time) that the fibroid tumors were the cause of being unable to conceive.

Another year passed. By the summer of 2005, we still hadn't become pregnant. For my yearly ob-gyn appointment, I requested to be seen by another physician. The new doctor confirmed the previous physician's findings and recommended we exercise patience; conception would happen once my body fully healed from the surgery. His findings were no comfort, and due to my age (I was in my thirties at this point), I requested a repeat of the dye test of my fallopian tubes to ensure there was still no blockage. The new test yielded the same result. I felt comfortable letting nature take its course.

The First Rejection

In the fall of 2005, I took a position that required me to travel to another state and return home each weekend. My husband and I weren't taking precautions to prevent pregnancy, and we believed that it would eventually happen. When questions came from well-intentioned family and friends about why we didn't have children, we explained that we were focused on our careers and education at that point, though we were confident we would soon be pregnant. These questions made me wonder if something else was wrong, but I dismissed my concerns because my ob-gyn said there was no reason we hadn't become pregnant.

Three months into my new job, I returned home one weekend and began experiencing a nagging pain in my lower-right abdomen. Initially, I concluded that the pain was from inadvertently lifting too much. From Friday to Sunday, the pain persisted. I took some over-the-counter medication. My husband tried to convince me to stay home and go to the doctor. I didn't take his advice and proceeded with my weekly Sunday travels.

On Monday morning, the pain increased significantly. By midday, the pain was more than I could tolerate and forced me to go to a local emergency room. The doctor pressed on my right side to evaluate how uncomfortable the pressure made me feel. When I winced in pain, he asked me a battery of questions about how long I'd been in pain, my level of discomfort, and if I'd had any problems with my appendix. Finally, he asked if I was pregnant and instructed me to take a pregnancy test. After waiting for what seemed like an eternity, he confirmed the result: I was pregnant!

Naïve as I was about pain during pregnancy, aside from brief mentions of miscarriages in my family, I called my husband and several close family members and told them that I was finally pregnant and in the hospital with some related pain. They reassured me to stay calm and rest. None of these important people in my life gave me any indication that I should worry.

When the doctor returned, he said he was concerned about the pain and suggested that I return home to see my own ob-gyn. He believed the pregnancy was ectopic, a condition that occurs in about one out of every fifty pregnancies when the fertilized egg implants itself in the fallopian tube or another location outside of the uterus.

This news caused mixed emotions. I was happy that we'd achieved pregnancy, but I was also worried that something was terribly wrong. I tried to remain optimistic and asked about the possibility of the pregnancy being full term given the preliminary diagnosis. The doctor repeated that I should speak to my primary ob-gyn. His primary concern was for me to be seen immediately, as he didn't want to risk the fallopian tube bursting. If the pregnancy was indeed ectopic, we would need to terminate immediately because if the problem wasn't handled quickly, then I would jeopardize my life and future fertility.

Imagine, on the same day, in just a few hours, receiving the best and worst news ever. For what seemed like an eternity, we'd been trying to conceive and had finally done so, only to have that bright ray of hope jeopardized by the news that the pregnancy might not be viable. After leaving the emergency room, I called my doctor. I made flight arrangements to return home that evening so I could make my next-day appointment.

At my regular ob-gyn, I was whisked inside immediately for a battery of tests to evaluate my condition and determine next steps. Specifically, the pregnancy test was repeated, an ultrasound was performed to determine the location of the fertilized egg, my temperature and blood pressure were evaluated, and the doctor pressed on my right side to determine how sensitive I would be to pressure applied to that area.

After the tests, we waited anxiously to hear the results and tried to remain optimistic. The doctor returned to the room and explained that the pregnancy was ectopic. He proceeded to outline the next course of action. We were devastated. We could hardly process what the doctor was outlining for us. Seeing our reaction, he agreed to give my husband and me a few moments to decide what we would do, though we needed to decide that day.

Before leaving the room, the doctor summarized our options. These were surgery to remove the pregnancy or a medication called methotrexate. Choosing the medication would allow me to avoid another surgery, but it would require weekly blood work to determine if my human chorionic gonadotropin (HCG) levels were decreasing. A decrease in HCG would mean that the pregnancy was dissolving, and no further action would be needed. If the blood work indicated an increase or no decrease in HCG, then surgery would need to be considered.

Once the doctor departed, we discussed our options as rationally as we could. Before this experience, we truly believed that once we received a confirmed pregnancy test, we wouldn't have to worry. But we'd been terribly wrong.

We decided to go with the medication to dissolve the pregnancy. With this decision came the administration of methotrexate in my buttock area and information on what we should expect to follow: some cramping and potential spotting that would mimic a menstrual cycle.

After the appointment, we had to make difficult calls to the family and friends whom we'd told about our pregnancy. They said how sorry they were for our loss and said that we could always try again. Given the news we'd just received and our painful decision, that was the last thing we wanted to hear. Still, we thanked everyone and said we'd try again when we were given clearance. I felt like a complete failure and that I'd let my husband and my family down, and that I'd personally failed the unborn child who we would never know.

My body quickly responded to the methotrexate, and I began to experience the cramp-like symptoms soon after its administration. Several days later, I returned to the doctor for the first blood work to check HCG levels.

While there was a slight decrease, I was instructed to return the next week for another reading. The blood tests were repeated over numerous weeks until the results reached the level that indicated I was no longer pregnant. Once the doctor was satisfied with the HCG level, we scheduled an appointment to discuss our next steps on this parenthood journey.

REJECTION REPEATED

After the first loss, I never imagined that we'd continue to experience pregnancy difficulties. Family and friends who were trying to be helpful repeatedly stated that after the first pregnancy, subsequent pregnancies were easier, as the body tended to be more fertile. Armed with their advice, we had a follow-up appointment with my doctor to discuss when we would be able to try to conceive again. He recommended having two menstrual cycles following the first ectopic pregnancy and the methotrexate treatment. He agreed with our family's outlook, so we were optimistic about our future pregnancy outcomes.

By January 2006, I had another confirmed pregnancy. While the pregnancy wasn't ectopic, eight weeks into the pregnancy, I experienced what I learned to be a missed pregnancy (or miscarriage). The pregnancy began correctly, but my body ultimately rejected it. During this pregnancy, we didn't share any news with family, as we wanted everything confirmed with the doctor after the first pregnancy and the emotional toll of repeating what happened multiple times. Following the miscarriage, I was once again subjected to blood tests to monitor HCG levels to ensure the pregnancy was indeed dissolved.

Between 2006 and 2010, I endured repeated ectopic pregnancies and miscarriages. In total, I experienced seven lost pregnancies. Several of them ended with methotrexate.

An ectopic pregnancy in 2010 changed the course of our parenthood journey. Once again, to end the pregnancy, methotrexate was administered. I had made it to about the nine-week mark, and the medication to end the pregnancy was administered a bit later once the pregnancy was confirmed.

After the methotrexate, the cramping began like clockwork; this time, however, the pain was severe. In fact, it was so severe that I called out of work and informed my boss that I wouldn't be in the next day. Before the night was over, the cramping became so intense that it woke me up. I got up to go to the bathroom and tried to keep quiet so that I wouldn't wake my husband. Stepping off the bed, I stood up, and the pain was so bad that I cried out.

At that moment, I started bleeding profusely. I tried to make it to the bathroom to clean myself up and began to pass huge blood clots. The pain and bleeding were so intense that I ended up in a childlike pose on the bedroom floor, rocking myself to get the pain to stop. My husband carried me to the bathroom. He was so concerned that he called an ambulance to take me to the emergency room. I was hospitalized and couldn't return to work for four weeks.

After this ordeal, we met with the doctor again. The doctor informed us that we probably shouldn't try to get pregnant again on our own. He would refer us to an in vitro fertilization (IVF) specialist. He was confident that we would be successful through IVF, as we didn't seem to have a problem getting pregnant. He was also worried about my health if we continued trying to conceive naturally. With this referral, he advised us of the expense associated with IVF, though he expressed confidence that this was the way for us to successfully conceive.

My husband and I embraced the referral. After so many losses, we were desperate for answers and wanted to explore all options before accepting that we may never become parents. When conceiving naturally, my body had rejected each pregnancy between the six- to eight-week mark not once but seven times! What other choice did we have? By then, our choices were to consider adoption or IVF, so we accepted that we shouldn't try again to conceive naturally. We began our IVF journey to parenthood in 2011.

Acceptance

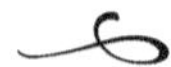

IVF Cycle #1

While excited about the potential to conceive using IVF, it was somewhat difficult to put aside the fact of conceiving naturally. I was supposed to be able to do this—I again questioned my womanhood and why this was happening to me. During this time, family, friends, and coworkers were conceiving and having children with ease. While I was happy for them, it was hard to process and accept. Although I knew it was the only viable option for us to explore, it was difficult to accept that my husband and I would need help getting pregnant. Coupled with the expense of the procedure, IVF was one of the biggest decisions of our lives. We accepted our fate and began the conversations to find out more on what to expect from the process.

The first appointment at the IVF clinic proved fruitful. My medical records were sent over from the ob-gyn's office before the visit, and the fertility doctor was able to evaluate our situation. During the first visit, he determined that he concurred with the assessment of the ob-gyn and urged us not to conceive naturally. Since we didn't have a problem getting pregnant, he felt half the battle was conquered. The fertility doctor also questioned the number of prior surgeries I'd had and concluded that there may be scar tissue from the surgeries that might have been the reason for the repeated ectopic pregnancies and miscarriages. At the end of the appointment, he recommended a repeat of the dye test to evaluate the condition of my fallopian tubes and an evaluation of my uterus to assess my candidacy for IVF. We worked with the scheduling staff, and appointments were made to conduct these tests in a future visit later that week.

I returned to the IVF clinic a few days later for the tests. First, my uterus was evaluated and found to be in good condition; however, the fibroid tumors had returned. The dye test was conducted to evaluate the condition of my tubes, and while the dye flowed through each of the tubes, the right tube did not release all of the dye, which led the fertility doctor to conclude that my tubes were not in great shape after all. Once the tests were conducted, I got dressed to prepare to listen to the full debrief of the appointment. During the debrief, the fertility doctor encouraged us to consider the following options prior to proceeding with a round of IVF to improve our chances of conceiving:

- Remove my tubes—there was a chance that the pregnancy would be ectopic because even with IVF, ectopic pregnancies can still occur.
- Remove the fibroid tumors—the location of the tumors could make it difficult to place the future fertilized embryo in the correct place.

The doctor also informed us that we could choose to move forward with the IVF cycle without the recommendations because we may get lucky on the first try and the surgical options could be avoided. We considered our options, and I discussed with my husband how I felt about removing my tubes. While they had proven to be of no use to me, removing a major part of my reproductive system was a huge point to consider. We decided to forego the surgeries and proceed with the IVF. After all, we were always able to conceive, and the IVF process would just ensure that the pregnancy would situate itself in the correct place.

To begin the IVF, we had to go to education classes to learn what to expect from the process. During the class, we were provided a schedule to guide the process from beginning to end. The most intimidating part of the process, in my opinion, was the numerous medications that I would need to administer to myself to produce eggs that would be removed and later fertilized with my husband's sperm. This would eventually lead to embryos that would be implanted. If I responded well to the medications and the egg retrieval, then all would be well—or so we thought.

The medications prescribed to allow my body to produce eggs seemed to agree with me, and I responded well. After self-administering the medications, I was able to produce eggs. The doctor was able to retrieve fifteen of them. Of those fifteen, seven were fertilized and proved to be good enough for the IVF round. My husband and I were excited that things went so well. To prepare for embryo implantation during IVF, I went to the doctor's office multiple times to determine if the lining of the uterus was the right length so that the embryo can be placed in the correct environment to lead to a confirmed pregnancy. Typically, the fertility clinic will implant one or more embryos to maximize success. Before doing so, the fertility doctor will discuss the number of embryos a couple is willing to implant because in vitro can lead to multiple births. Also, prior to the fertility doctor actually implanting the embryo(s), the fertility doctor will often do a trial run to ensure that they implant the embryo(s) in the correct place.

Prior to the doctor implanting the embryos, I had to drink water to fill my bladder so the doctor could see where to implant the embryos. During the test run, the doctor seemed to be having difficulties and outlined that my uterus was tilted, which made access difficult; however, he was sure that he would be able to implant the two embryos for this IVF round. When the doctor began to implant the embryos, we were able to watch via ultrasound the embryos being implanted in my uterus. We thought it was an awesome experience to actually see when you may have possibly conceived on an ultrasound!

Following the procedure, I had to lie with my legs in the stirrups for twenty minutes before departing for home. When I got up to leave, I felt liquid run down my leg and told the nurse that I was concerned something was not right. She assured me that the experience was normal because of my bladder being full and because of the procedure. The nurse said that I should not be concerned about the embryos falling out and to resume normal activities. Following that appointment, my husband and I went to church, as the procedure took place on a Sunday. We would return to the clinic in fourteen days for a pregnancy test to hopefully confirm the pregnancy. We were instructed to resist the urge of conducting a home pregnancy test, which could give an erroneous reading because of the IVF medications.

We returned to the clinic fourteen days later as instructed for the pregnancy test. The pregnancy test conducted was a blood test, which is the most accurate when undergoing IVF. Unfortunately, our excitement was dashed, as the pregnancy test confirmed that we were not pregnant. We were heartbroken and asked direct questions about the embryo transfer and voiced our concerns directly to the doctor. The fertility doctor confirmed that he had difficulties with the embryo transfer, but he assured us that he had indeed planted the embryos in the correct place despite those difficulties. He also said we still had five frozen embryos and we could try again as that was covered in the original cost of the cycle. But he urged us to reconsider removing my tubes and the fibroids to maximize success.

After much discussion, we decided that I would have laparoscopic surgery to remove the fibroid tumors; however, I was still adamant about not wanting to remove my tubes. As we were removing the fibroids, it would be six months before we would be able to undergo IVF again. A few weeks after the first IVF procedure, my laparoscopic surgery was performed by my IVF doctor. I was able to go home the day of the surgery and was back to my normal routine in about three weeks.

IVF Cycle #2

At the beginning of 2012, we started the second IVF cycle. This IVF round was much easier on me than the first because I did not have to produce eggs since we were going to use two of the frozen embryos from the last IVF cycle. I still had to give myself injections to thicken my uterine lining to prepare for the transfer and subsequent medications until a confirmed pregnancy test. We were really hopeful things would work this cycle because the fibroids were removed.

Once again, the doctor conducted his trial run prior to the embryo transfer and experienced difficulties with placement. I expressed my concern and pushed for him to ensure that he could place the embryos in the correct place without struggling to do so. After a few trial runs, he was able to adjust the technique enough without demonstrating the earlier struggle. An hour or so later, the last of the embryos for this IVF round would be implanted. We only had three of the remaining five embryos survive the thawing process. So, instead of two embryos being implanted, we opted to go with three, fully realizing the potential of multiple births. Given the expense and our pregnancy struggles, we figured multiple births in one pregnancy and avoiding another IVF round would be totally worth it in the end.

Fourteen days later, we returned to the doctor's office for a pregnancy test. This time, however, I chose to conduct a pregnancy test at home prior to the one at the doctor's office. While conducting home pregnancy tests are not recommended while undergoing this process, my anxiety and excitement got the better of me. The home pregnancy test yielded that we had not conceived. My husband, trying to remain optimistic, communicated that the home pregnancy test may be wrong and that I should adhere to the instructions given regarding the pregnancy test. At the doctor's office, the blood test was run to determine pregnancy success. The home pregnancy test was confirmed to be true; we had not conceived with this IVF round. Given that we had used all the embryos, where were we to turn next?

Upon receiving the pregnancy results, we had another consult with the IVF doctor. He explained that there was no reason why we had not conceived. He urged us to pursue another IVF round. We were extremely disappointed with the outcomes of the IVF rounds and communicated that we would consider it, though we thought that it might be highly unlikely given the cost. The doctor urged us not to give up and proceeded to give us information on adoption to consider.

While we took the adoption information and investigated the possibility, private adoption was just as expensive as another IVF round. The thought of getting attached to a child and then the birth parents having the opportunity to claim the child as their own deterred us from pursuing the adoption route. When pursuing adoption, there is a window of time where the birth parents can change their mind. Usually the time allowed is a year before the adoption can be finalized. Since we were unsuccessful conceiving at the current IVF clinic, we decided to try another fertility clinic before giving up on this journey.

IVF Clinic #2

Prior to the consult with the second IVF clinic, I began to experience excruciating abdomen pain and difficulty lying flat. These symptoms persisted for about five days until I finally acquiesced and went to urgent care to determine the cause of the pain. During this time, I had difficulty keeping food down, and there was a constant burning sensation in my upper stomach and chest. The physician's assistant who evaluated my symptoms concluded that it was my gallbladder and immediately referred me to a radiology clinic for further evaluation. Upon examination, it was confirmed that my gallbladder was infected and would need to be removed laparoscopically.

When I questioned the doctor on the gallbladder issue, he outlined that the IVF medications I had taken caused my gallbladder to become infected, and there was no other recourse than surgery. This was not news I wanted to hear given that I had fibroids removed before the last IVF round, and the doctor would be using the same entry points to remove my gallbladder laparoscopically. These entry points are permanent reminders of the struggles we had with trying to conceive. This procedure would deter any progress with setting an appointment with a fertility doctor at the new IVF clinic. It would be another two to three months before we had a consult with the new IVF clinic to ensure I was totally healed from the surgery.

After healing from the gallbladder surgery, we went for our consult with the IVF doctor at the second clinic. While healing, I had researched the clinic's success rates and each of its respective fertility doctors. The research yielded that the female fertility doctor had the highest success rates, and we pressed to see her given all we had been through in our prior IVF rounds. We were informed that it was not guaranteed that we would see the same doctor throughout the process; however, we were adamant that due to our prior experiences, we were only comfortable seeing one particular physician throughout the process. Reluctantly, the clinic listened to our request, and we were seen by one fertility doctor throughout the IVF process.

Upon seeing the desired fertility doctor, a battery of questions was asked followed by a final question on the possibility of being pregnant. While my husband and I had not been taking any precautions to prevent pregnancy, the fertility doctor wanted to conduct a pregnancy test prior to us beginning the IVF round. Surprisingly, the pregnancy test came back positive! While ecstatic with the result, we remained subdued with the news given our prior confirmed pregnancies. Upon conducting an ultrasound to determine the pregnancy's location (as our previous pregnancies were ectopic or early miscarriages), it was determined that I was approximately eight weeks pregnant and that this pregnancy was not viable, as it was also determined to be an early miscarriage. Upon receiving this news, devastation and defeat set in once again. The new fertility doctor recommended a procedure called dilation and curettage (D and C) to remove the pregnancy. The procedure was scheduled the following day and was extremely painful to endure.

Prior to beginning the IVF round, the fertility doctor recommended removing my tubes as defective tubes can sometimes cause difficulty with a successful IVF cycle. Given the expense, I made the difficult decision to remove my tubes, eliminating any possibility of us being able to conceive naturally. While I knew this was the best option, I was emotionally devastated with the knowledge that I would always need assistance to conceive. The new fertility doctor would eventually use the same laparoscopic entry points from the prior fibroid and gallbladder surgeries to remove my fallopian tubes. She communicated that it would be about six to eight weeks before we could begin the IVF process.

Since we needed to go through the entire IVF process of producing eggs to be fertilized with my husband's sperm, this IVF round was a bit more taxing on me both emotionally and physically. On the egg-retrieval day, the fertility clinic was able to retrieve approximately eight eggs of which six were determined to be viable and successfully fertilized. The fertility doctor would later recommend that three of the six be implanted for a greater success rate. We agreed with the recommendation and prayed for a positive pregnancy test. However, it was not meant to be. Upon returning to the clinic to confirm the pregnancy, the pregnancy test yielded a negative result. We were yet again not successful.

At this point, our finances were running low, as was our optimism that we would become parents. My husband communicated to me that he was happy with it just being the two of us, but I was not ready to accept defeat. We still had three frozen embryos, and to me that meant there was still a possibility. By this point, it was late 2012, and I did not want to risk not being successful with IVF any longer. I started to do more research on another IVF clinic and what else I could do to increase our odds of succeeding. We did not return to this clinic but instead chose to go to the top clinic in our area to pursue next steps. It would be a bit costlier but hopefully well worth it in the end.

IVF Clinic #3

In deciding to go to the third IVF clinic, we would exhaust our savings, including borrowing from a 401(k) retirement account to pay for the treatment. We decided to exhaust our savings to prevent another financed loan expense. This would be the last chance at conception, and we had to decide at this point that we would not pursue the parenthood journey any longer if we were not successful.

Given that we were not going to return to the second IVF clinic, we had the three remaining frozen embryos transferred to the third clinic. The research conducted on the third clinic proved promising. Success rates were better than the two clinics we had been to in our prior IVF rounds. We met with the top fertility doctor at the clinic for the original consult, where I had to rehash our pregnancy struggles and the reason we were seeing him at this point in time. Upon listening to my pregnancy history and realizing that I no longer had my fallopian tubes, he communicated that his assessment yielded that I did not need to have the tubes removed, and he wished that I had seen him prior to their removal, as the clinic was known for its success with a tubal-repair procedure. Since this was no longer an option, the IVF discussion began, and we determined the next steps. While the three remaining embryos were transferred from the second clinic, the fertility doctor recommended that we pursue a full IVF round in case the frozen embryos were not viable. Additionally, he was not enthused about using the embryos from the other clinic, as he was not sure of the process they used, which could jeopardize our success rate.

During the first visit, we communicated the difficulties other fertility doctors experienced with the embryo transfers due to my uterus being tilted. The doctor communicated he had experience and success with these situations and outlined that he would conduct a test run that same day to see if he would experience difficulty with embryo placement. We were amazed with the ease he had with the trial run, and he noted he would conduct another prior to the actual transfer. He surmised that our failure was not due to the IVF procedures but the techniques the previous IVF doctors had used with the embryo transfer. He was confident we would successfully conceive if we settled on using him as our IVF doctor. We left the doctor's office that day feeling optimistic about the potential of becoming parents and settled on moving forward with the fertility doctor at the third clinic.

Prior to moving forward with the next IVF round, I began to change some daily habits to maximize IVF success, since we had not been successful in other rounds. I changed my eating habits and started to eat organic foods and eliminated certain foods from my diet. Before the IVF cycle, I decided to undergo a cleanse to ensure I was in perfect condition to receive and nurture the future life I would eventually grow inside me. Additionally, I started attending regular acupuncture sessions to help my mental and physical well-being. The acupuncturist conducted specific treatments focused on maximizing fertility. Also, attending therapy prior to undergoing this IVF cycle was instrumental to success, because I needed to be mentally prepared for whatever would come and accept any consequences. It was through therapy that I realized that I had not truly grieved each of my pregnancy losses/unsuccessful pregnancies and discovered I had a lot of resentment against myself. I resented myself as I felt I was not able to do the one thing that most women are able to achieve seamlessly. In addition, I felt that I had failed my husband.

Feeling truly prepared to undergo the next IVF cycle, we called the IVF doctor and began the process. In January 2013, we were blessed to discover that the IVF procedure was successful, and we received a positive pregnancy result! The pregnancy was proceeding nicely, and the baby was developing as it should. We found out in May that the baby was a girl, and we were overjoyed with the possibility of welcoming her into the world in November of that year.

As we prepared for the birth of our baby girl, whom we would name Erin Janelle, I was also caring for my mom, who had raised me. She had battled heart issues, sarcoidosis, and pulmonary hypertension for over fifteen years. Her fight for life was significant; she was in intensive care from October 2012 through May 2013. I had the opportunity to let her know we were pregnant, and she was overjoyed for us. But she would never know our baby girl, because in May 2013, she passed from complications of her illness. It was a devastating time, because one of the people who loved me like no other was no longer with me. Her death hit me hard; however, I tried to remain strong because the baby would be born in her birthday month, November, which I took as confirmation that this pregnancy was meant to be.

Less than a month after my mom passed, more devastation knocked at my door. The date was June 4, 2013. My life would never be the same. I was approximately eighteen weeks pregnant and went to the restroom to urinate, or so I thought. While using the restroom, I noticed a bulging sac and became so alarmed that I called out to my husband. Not knowing what to do, we immediately went to the closest emergency room to get a diagnosis while hoping and praying that nothing was happening to the baby. Upon examination from the emergency-room doctor, he immediately transferred me to the hospital, where I could be seen by the ob-gyn who had been caring for me since the successful pregnancy.

After being seen by the ob-gyn, it was confirmed that my amniotic sac had burst and labor was imminent. Confused by this news, we asked a plethora of questions on what that meant and why it happened. We were told that my cervix gave way and became open, a rare condition that indicated to my pregnant body that it was time to give birth. Also, the ob-gyn outlined that while the baby seemed fine at that moment, if born at eighteen weeks, she would not survive. I was clearly pregnant to everyone in my life, and to go through the process of losing this baby so publicly was devastating.

Given that birth was imminent, and as the baby could not survive without an amniotic sac, I was whisked off to labor and delivery, the same floor where women were having healthy and live babies. About six hours after seeing the ob-gyn, the contractions began, and I was told that the more frequent they became, the closer the baby was to being born. Imagine pushing for several hours to deliver a baby who lived only four hours and saying good-bye to her in the same breath. I once again felt like a failure and that my body refused to carry the life that was growing inside me. I was the reason Erin was no longer with us. The ob-gyn outlined that the correct term for this phenomenon was an "incompetent cervix." At the time, I felt it was the perfect name for what I was feeling: incompetent as a woman.

Following a birth, a woman must also deliver the placenta. This process is painful and if not passed naturally, the placenta must be removed surgically. After delivering Erin, the doctor tried for hours to remove the placenta; however, she was not successful, and I was whisked off to have it removed surgically. As the doctor proceeded to remove the placenta, I began hemorrhaging to the point of needing a blood transfusion. Imagine the position of my husband at the time, who had just lost his first live child and who was also possibly on the brink of losing his wife. After stabilizing me, the doctor was successful in removing the placenta. Several days later, I was sent home to recover and scheduled for a follow-up with the ob-gyn.

The follow-up appointment after delivering Erin was one of the most difficult appointments of my life. There were women there who'd had healthy babies around the same time we lost her. During the appointment, I had difficulty holding myself together and broke down in uncontrollable tears at the doctor's office. After pulling myself together, an examination was conducted, and we met with the doctor for the required follow-up. She expressed sympathy for our loss since she knew all we had gone through to achieve pregnancy. Also, she communicated that should we decide to try again, she would strongly recommend a cerclage at eighteen weeks to help keep my cervix closed for the reminder of the next pregnancy.

I was so angry and devastated at this point that I could not even consider moving forward with the parenthood journey. Frankly, I felt I could not endure any more pain and loss; life was not fair to have taken so much from me, from us in such a short time. I had lost my mom, and less than one month later, I had lost the promise of a child. I was totally crushed. Since my ob-gyn office and the fertility clinic were partners, the fertility doctor heard about the loss and had his assistant reach out to us to begin the discussion of trying again. Before any of this could happen, I really needed to process and seek therapy to heal. After a couple of months, while hesitant, we moved forward with another IVF round, understanding that if we were successful, a vaginal cerclage would be placed to prevent my cervix from opening. The IVF doctor who was successful with the pregnancy of Erin would conduct the next IVF.

Hope

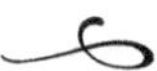

After losing Erin and my mom, I learned that I had the strength to endure devastating loss and that I could recover with therapy, prayer, and nourishing myself both physically and mentally. With this revelation came the determination to succeed on the parenthood journey, as we had come so close with Erin. I was hopeful that we would be successful because we now knew everything that had prohibited us from becoming parents before—or so we thought. We decided to move forward with another IVF round, expecting to receive the news that we had conceived. By October 2013, I was pregnant with our second child, optimistic that all would be well and expecting the cerclage to be placed around week eighteen or nineteen of the pregnancy.

During this pregnancy, the fertility doctor recommended that I take progesterone injections to help support the pregnancy. I took the progesterone shots each night, and the pregnancy progressed well. There seemed to be no complications, and the cerclage was placed at week nineteen of the pregnancy. The follow-up appointment after the cerclage placement was promising, and I progressed to week twenty-three of the pregnancy. I had been taking it easy this pregnancy and thought we were well on our way to a successful birth because I was so far along. Then tragedy struck again.

In order for medical professionals to intervene with a pregnancy, a woman must make it to the twenty-fifth week of pregnancy. Around week twenty-three, I began to experience some complications. We had gone to the doctor for a checkup, and during the ultrasound examination, the technician communicated that all was well with the baby (a girl), but she wanted the doctor to examine me. While she tried to reassure me, we were immediately alarmed given all we had been through on our parenthood journey. Upon examination by the doctor, it was discovered that despite the cerclage placement, my cervix was opening again, causing my body to think that it was time to deliver the baby. I was placed immediately on bedrest and was required to return to the doctor's office for a more comprehensive exam the next day.

Upon returning to the doctor, he conducted a test to see if the baby was doing well. She (whom we named Peyton Elise Smith) seemed to be thriving; however, the doctor was concerned that my cervix appeared more open than the day before and insisted we consider removing the cerclage because if I went into labor with the cerclage, it would rip the vaginal area. We were so close to twenty-five weeks, and if I could just hold on and not go into labor, all would be well. Since we ultimately decided not to remove the cerclage, I was required to return to the doctor's office every other day so that my cervix could be examined. We were instructed that if contractions started, I was to go to the maternity ward immediately so the cerclage could be removed and the baby delivered.

I remained on bedrest through week twenty-three and seemed to be holding on with no change in my cervix opening. On the first day of week twenty-four, I began to experience minor contractions, but I kept that to myself, as I really wanted to hold on as long as I could to increase the chances that Peyton would survive. By the next day, I could not hide that I was having contractions. We called the doctor's office, and he arranged for us to have a quick check-in at the nearby hospital. This appointment was the beginning of the end of my pregnancy with Peyton.

Visiting the nearby partnering hospital to see the supposed expert in these situations was terrible on all accounts. The doctor who saw us in labor and delivery was rude, insensitive, and refused to listen to what I was explaining was happening with the pregnancy. He wanted to remove the cerclage immediately without a discussion to determine or explore other alternatives. Since we were so close to the twenty-fifth week, we researched and saw cases of women in my situation being turned almost upside-down to relieve the pressure from the cervix with insertions of progesterone to the vaginal area to eliminate the contractions. Turning a woman upside down and inserting progesterone in the vagina are tactics used to stop early labor. This solution we thought would give us a better chance of bringing Peyton home. The doctor became combative and dismissive to the point that my husband checked me out of the hospital that night. We ended up at another hospital that would give us hope of bringing Peyton home.

We decided to go to this doctor as my best friend recommended him and he was a renowned expert in his field. At the hospital, we were immediately seen by the new physician, who examined me and started a course of action to save the baby. Amazingly, the course of action taken was what we were trying to get the other doctor to consider. This doctor was concerned about the consistency of the contractions and informed us that if they did not subside, the cerclage would need to be removed. But he would do everything he could to ensure that the baby was not born until week twenty-five.

Since he knew the baby would be born early, he told us that if I could hold on until week twenty-five, they would begin to administer medication to help develop her lungs so that she would be able to breath on her own once born. The doctor and his staff kept a constant watch over me, and later that night, the contractions subsided. Once they subsided, we were moved into a room on the maternity ward, where they tilted my bed at an angle that situated me almost upside down. If I could hold on through the night without contractions, my chances of making it to week twenty-five would be greatly increased.

After we made it through the night, we began to relax just a bit. Around midday on February 13, 2014, the contractions started again, and the doctor was called immediately. After examination, he informed us that the cerclage needed to be removed because I would risk too much damage if it ripped. Since the danger to myself was increasing, we had no other choice but to allow the cerclage to be removed. After its removal, I remained in the upside-down position to see how long we could hold on without the cerclage.

While going through all this, we began to see snow falling outside the window. We got so much snow! It was a good thing that I was actually in the hospital because had this happened at home during a snowstorm, things would have ended much differently. I may have not survived, and any chance of parenthood would have been forever lost. The contractions once again subsided; however, later that night, they started again, and I knew Peyton would be born at any time.

The nurse called the doctor, and moments later I was whisked to labor and delivery to begin the process of having Peyton. She was born on February 14, 2014. She was born on the right day—Valentine's Day—and at that moment, we poured all the love we could into her. We were informed that if she could make if through the night, there would be a high likelihood that she would survive, despite being born weeks early. During this time, we rocked and held her, and she smiled and reacted to our voices.

Eight hours later, we all fell asleep. When we woke up, Peyton's time had ended. Since she had lived several hours, we had to go through the process of signing paperwork for her birth certificate. While she was no longer with us, there would forever be physical proof that she once lived. During my pregnancy with Erin, we were not given this opportunity because Erin was born much earlier.

During my pregnancy with Peyton, I constantly craved Cuties® Mandarins. The entire time I was in the hospital, I ate them like they were going out of style. By the time that I delivered her, there was only one left. When we looked at the last orange after Peyton's delivery and passing, a small heart had formed on the orange. We took that as a sign that Peyton knew we loved her and that it was okay to let her go. We were devastated and did not know in which direction to turn after another gut-wrenching loss.

The positive thing that happened after Peyton's birth was the doctor who delivered and treated me at the hospital. This doctor was known for placing a different type of cerclage that was guaranteed to result in a full-term pregnancy. He informed us that if we considered pregnancy again, he would like for us to see him prior to the pregnancy, and he would place a cerclage that could be permanent or removed at the time of delivery. The caveat to this cerclage is that I would not be able to deliver vaginally, and it would need to be placed prior to conception.

It would be a couple of months before we could even fathom pursuing another IVF round, but we eventually did. I had a transvaginal cervicoisthmic cerclage (TVCIC) placed prior to beginning the IVF cycle to ensure success. Doing so gave me and my husband hope that this time we would bring a baby home should we conceive.

Endure

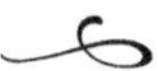

A TVCIC is a type of cerclage that is less common than the traditional cerclage and has greater success rates. Prior to undergoing the procedure to have it placed, a lot of research was conducted to help gauge success rates. I was surprised to see that there were specific closed groups one could join online and to see the number of women who had endured a loss or two because of incompetent cervix issues and had the TVCIC cerclage placed to bring home a bundle of joy.

At this point, we had endured so much pregnancy loss that we decided this IVF cycle would be our last. Whether or not we were successful, we had been through enough, and it was time for the journey to end. In August 2014, I started my last and final IVF cycle with the remaining frozen embryos. Much like the previous cycles, I continued with acupuncture and underwent a cleanse with clean eating to ensure conception. Multiple eggs were implanted, and once again at the end of the IVF cycle, we would wait fourteen days before a pregnancy could be confirmed.

This IVF round, I did not conduct a home pregnancy test prior to visiting the IVF clinic to confirm the pregnancy. All I could do was pray and nourish myself mentally and physically to endure to the end. When we returned to the doctor's office to take the pregnancy test, we were pleased again to learn that we were expecting! We received this news in October 2014 and were informed that we should expect delivery of this child in April 2015. A week later, I participated in my commencement celebration for my doctorate in educational leadership.

Since the doctor who placed the TVCIC was the best doctor in the area, we entrusted my pregnancy care to him. Plus he had been so kind and understanding with my last delivery that it was a no-brainer to partner with him. In most cases, patients seeing ob-gyn physicians must see all doctors in the practice during a pregnancy. This doctor ensured that at each appointment, he would be the one examining me, and he assured me that we would bring this baby home. For this pregnancy, I was required to see the doctor biweekly through week eighteen, and once we hit the twenty-fourth week, the visits would be weekly.

While the doctor was sure that all would be well and that these appointments were not a true necessity, given what we had been through, he listened to my desire to be seen more frequently, and he accommodated my requests. This doctor was a true blessing to me during my pregnancy. Any worry was heard, and he even allowed me to have his cell phone number to text him if there were ever any complications.

During week eighteen of the pregnancy, I was at work and went to the restroom and was alarmed to see that I had started spotting. I texted the doctor who instructed me to come into the office immediately. I informed my boss that I needed to leave early because I was experiencing complications and needed to report to the doctor. At his office, the doctor asked me a series of questions to gauge the problem and asked me to explain what I thought was going on to better customize my care in this situation. I clearly remember the doctor stating that I knew my body best given our prior losses. It was a relief to have someone who would advocate for me during a pregnancy.

After much discussion, it was determined that all was well, but given that I had stopped using the progesterone injections, it was just dried blood that was passing and not due to not using the medication. However, at my urging, the doctor had me resume the progesterone injections and shots until week twenty-five of the pregnancy. Following this pregnancy scare, there were no more issues. When we reached the twenty-five-week gestational mark with the pregnancy, we were so thrilled. Even if the baby came early, we would be bringing our baby (a boy) home!

At the twenty-fifth week, the doctor began discussing scheduling the cesarean-section delivery date. We determined at that time that I would deliver the baby boy at week thirty-eight of pregnancy to ensure that contractions would not begin. On April 21, 2015, Ethan James Smith was born healthy at six pounds and nine ounces! It took a moment to process, but all we had endured led us to welcoming this baby boy into the world.

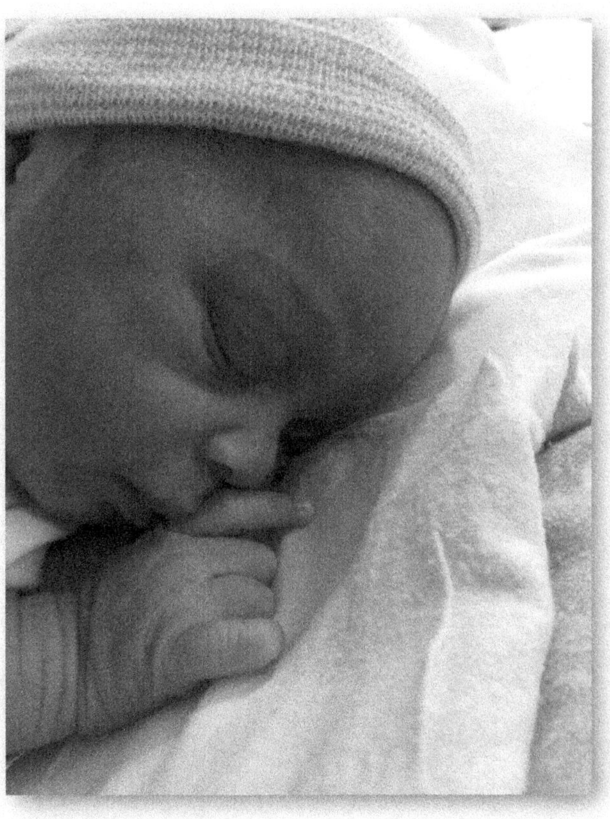

Five Steps to Moving Forward

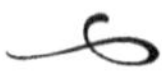

1. Build Endurance

The fertility journey requires endurance. At times, you will feel defeated because the process is more difficult than you thought or because you have hit another roadblock. During those times, it is important to have a meditation routine. Allow yourself to go to your quiet place where you can see yourself experiencing your parenthood dream. When you allow yourself to do so, you gain strength so that you can keep moving forward to your established goal.

Visualizing your dream helps you reach your ultimate destiny. Learning to visualize allows you to formulate a plan with specific goals. Vision exists to allow you to set goals to get where you are destined to be. Without vison, life is meaningless. Since your dream may have been deferred for some time, and you want to avoid making your heart sick, seeing yourself where you want to be helps your heart stay open.

As you build endurance, you will be tested and tried. Somedays, you will feel like the sun is shining in your favor, and on other days you may receive some devastating news that causes you to feel like you are engulfed in darkness. You will go through times where it may seem like you take a few steps forward and multiple steps back, which may cause fear to enter the picture. Do not let fear set in, as all things associated with fear provide a warped sense of reality and can take you off course and move you from a positive position.

Building endurance requires reflection. Evaluate your experiences to determine successes as well as situations that have delayed you on the fertility journey. It is important to reflect, but be careful not to get stuck in the past where you experienced a disappointment or heartbreak. Getting stuck in the past produces negative emotions and may slow the progress of the fertility journey. Reflection ultimately prepares you for the next step: therapy.

As you build endurance, you need to surround yourself with positive influences. If you try to build endurance alone, you will FAIL:

- **F**eel
- **A**lone
- **I**solated
- **L**onely

Positive influences provide the encouragement and hope you will need, no matter how short or long your journey has been. Those influences come in many forms: your spouse, close friends and family, written affirmations, quotes, songs, poems, prayers, and even self-encouragement. Adopt one or more of these positive influences, and you can find the strength to keep going. The positive influences help you as you hear or experience "no" and provide you an avenue to see delays as avenues that get you closer to your parenthood promise.

Remember, everything that happens on this journey assists you with arriving at new revelations and positions. Much like an athlete, endurance is important to completing your personal journey. You are running an unknown race, and without endurance, you quit and may not experience a future blessing.

2. Attend Therapy

Therapy is critical to the fertility journey. Overall, therapy helps you to

- be thankful in your current situation,
- heal your brokenness,
- express your feelings openly,

- alter negative thinking and feelings of depression,
- push through the challenging parenthood journey, and
- move on from the disappointment of yesterday, and focus on the future "yes."

Most importantly, therapy helps you heal your brokenness and can assist with you determining when you will end your fertility journey. Frankly, closure is needed after each loss and disappointment. Therapy provides perspective and allows you to stop blaming yourself for fertility difficulties or lost pregnancy. Therapy can serve as a positive influence and can come in many forms, such as groups (online and in-person), blogs, journaling, or creating a charity or foundation.

When in therapy, you are with a neutral party, which allows you to be totally open with what you are going through. Being around this neutral party allows you to express your true feelings without judgement and the worry of hurting those closest to you who have been with you on this journey. Therapy builds endurance, but it also prepares you for your next step: healing.

In therapy, you have the opportunity to process your cloudy days, heartbreak, depression, and hopes. As you process each of these in therapy, you will begin to forgive yourself, as on this journey, you begin to resent yourself for being unable to easily achieve parenthood like others around you. Forgiveness is the window that opens your heart. Without forgiveness, your heart becomes hard, and you close yourself (and your heart) to new possibilities.

3. START HEALING

When experiencing fertility struggles, you need to heal brokenness, heartbreaks, losses, and disappointments. Healing does not mean that you totally forget about your journey or the pain, losses, or disappointments you endured. Healing allows you to look back and see that you held strong and endured without becoming bitter. As the healing process takes root, your heart opens to new possibilities and future promises.

Without healing, you are unable to truly celebrate when others are prospering on the fertility journey while you continue to struggle. If you find it difficult to express happiness for others, it is a clear signal that you are harboring resentment and anger. During this time, it is important to remember that everything that is happening on the fertility journey is assisting you with new revelations and positions. It is okay to question why you continue to experience disappointments. As you heal, you are able to turn the "why" into action to get you to where you want to be or where you have accepted you are in this journey.

Healing looks different for everyone and may not be what you expect. For some, it is building a platform that helps others, taking a different path to obtain the parenthood dream (adoption, IVF, fertility treatments), or ending the journey. We each must allow healing to occur in the way that brings us the most comfort. There are many forms of healing, and acceptance is important.

Acceptance gives you your new position and allows you to begin or end your journey on your own terms. The new position with acceptance is being okay with not realizing the dream on your planned path or not traveling the path that society has painted as appropriate. As you heal, you will be okay with accepting that you may have to let go of a prior dream of "family" and can thrive with how you have decided to achieve or forego parenthood.

The last two steps in this process will not happen without healing: advocacy and nourishment. As you begin to heal, you are able to reflect on your experiences and research appropriate avenues that will inform the next steps in your journey.

There are many benefits to healing. The most helpful include the following:

- Helping to establish peace and acceptance
- Informing expectations and decisions
- Altering thinking and perceptions
- Prioritizing love over bitterness
- Eliminating feelings of jealousy

4. Be Your Own Advocate

Being your own advocate is the best thing you can do for yourself on this journey. As you experience fertility difficulties, you become intimately aware of your body and medical needs. Since you develop such a keen body awareness, it will be important to surround yourself with the appropriate professionals who will be open to listening to your needs and honoring your requests. Study your own medical records so you become well versed in the fertility language and, ultimately, your own needs.

To be an effective advocate, you must do the following:

- Pay attention to all details (feelings, medical records, case studies that are similar to what you are going through, past experiences on the journey).
- Develop a medical portfolio to keep track of each fertility experience, as a small detail can be the one thing keeping you from achieving your goals.
- Vet the medical professionals who are treating you, and seek multiple opinions.
- Openly report all that has happened to you. No one detail is too small. Now is not the time to withhold any information, no matter how embarrassing.
- Choose a competent medical professional who provides you with the honest details to help you reach your goals and clearly lays out all pros and cons.
- Assist your doctor with your care by following the prescribed course of action, and alert the doctor with negative or allergic reactions.
- Immediately tell your doctor when you have concerns about your care or treatment.
- Evaluate your care and progress. If you are being ignored or not making progress, make a decision to continue or immediately change medical professionals. Not doing so could be the difference between continuing to experience roadblocks and disappointments and taking the step that gets you to experience the parenthood dream.

Being your own advocate requires you to have or create a plan to help you reach your parenthood goals. Those going through the fertility journey need special care and attention. While there are typical textbook studies that dictate care, your situation may be unique enough to consider an alternative path. Research techniques based on what you have discovered that you need through lived experiences. The research you conduct allows you to become knowledgeable about what you have experienced or are currently going through. Advocacy helps you to have the appropriate and relevant conversations with those who care for you as you progress along the journey.

5. Nourish Yourself

The fertility journey is long and hard and requires you to nourish your mind, body, and soul. Your mind needs to be nourished because negative thoughts can take hold and become a roadblock. Nourishing your mind can be achieved by going to therapy, surrounding yourself with positive influences (see step 1), and seeking alternative therapies such as acupuncture. Mind nourishment must be a consistent ritual on this journey and is not typically done only once. Being consistent with nourishing your mind helps you build the endurance needed to persevere and positions you with achieving your set goals.

Body nourishment requires you to change your eating habits and exercise routines. On the fertility journey, you are preparing your body to accept and carry another human being. You will need to develop eating and exercise routines that are gentle to your body. All eating needs to be clean, meaning only organic foods should pass your lips and enter your body. Before beginning fertility treatments or when trying to conceive, cleanse your body of all toxins by detoxing. When you detox, you may discover there are some foods that are causing allergic reactions, which could be a reason you have not successfully achieved pregnancy. Once the negative food is revealed, eliminate this food entirely from your diet as you work to achieve parenthood.

Extreme exercise should be eliminated. Remember, your body is already stressed and strained because you are on this journey. The exercise you do should not be extreme, as you are already going through enough extreme measures to achieve pregnancy and parenthood. Adopt exercise that allows you to build endurance and can serve as a form of therapy, such as walking and yoga. These exercise types help you to maintain health and wellness and allow you to be kind to your body as you prepare for pregnancy on this parenthood journey. Exercises such as walking and yoga can also be continued once pregnancy is achieved.

Soul nourishment requires you to take care of your heart. To nourish your heart, you must heal (see step 3) your brokenness and feed yourself with positive influences. The details described in step 3 of this process lay the groundwork for consistent soul nourishment. Without feeding your soul with positivity, your progress toward reaching your goals will become derailed, as you will get discouraged and potentially give up before your scheduled time.

Ultimately you must nourish your mind, body, and soul to

- eliminate or keep negativity away;
- open your heart to receiving your parenthood dream;
- prepare your mind, body, and soul to undergo the necessary or chosen path;
- release mental, physical, and environmental toxins that may be delaying your progress;
- invite positive thinking and dreams;
- stop dwelling on past roadblocks or losses that hinder you from moving forward; and
- realize that everything that happens assists you with arriving at revelations and positions on the parenthood journey. Realizing this allows you to be kind to yourself and positions you for your ultimate goal of becoming a parent.

EPILOGUE

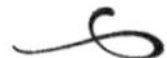

OUR JOURNEY TO PARENTHOOD WAS long and hard, with unexpected twists and turns. When we married in 2001, had anyone told me that our parenthood journey would have been this difficult, I would have dismissed the notion because we were programmed to believe that parenthood would happen so easily. I can honestly say that everything that happened on our parenthood journey helped me learn to expect, position, and endure so that we could bring Ethan home.

I learned a lot about myself and our marriage and maximized the five steps to success when experiencing the fertility issues that I outlined in the previous chapter. What I learned about myself is that I was and I am stronger than I ever thought I could be. Losing multiple children can break the strongest person. Also, experiencing multiple disappointments and rejections can cause depression and, at times, self-hatred. The most important thing I learned about my marriage is that my husband truly loves me and would stand by me through anything. As I was resenting myself, he was loving me in spite of the difficulties and assuring me that, through it all, we would be just fine.

There were a few close friends and family members who were our support system through this journey. These friends and family loved us through the losses, provided support and guidance, and ultimately rejoiced with us when we welcomed Ethan into the world. While going through the losses and the struggles to get pregnant was not enjoyable, quite frankly, everything that happened on this journey assisted me in arriving at new revelations and positions. Everything that I went through represents why Ethan is here today. We are so blessed to have him in our lives, and his being here reminds us that we endured.

I believe a part of me will always miss the babies I never got to know, but my heart is filled with joy because I have learned to accept the things I cannot change. Also, our struggles taught me some life lessons that assist me daily. Although the pain of the losses and struggles is real, I would not change anything because wishing for change would mean I would not have Ethan. At the end of the day, this fertility journey taught me three things:

1. I should expect blessings through difficult times.
2. I must position myself through constant prayer and the nourishment of my mind, body, and soul.
3. I will endure until the end because at the end of the journey is a rainbow of surprises.